Weight Loss Affirmations

Transform Your Mindset
and Achieve Your
Ideal Body

Melissa Fogel

Table Of Contents

Introduction

Conclusion

Introduction

John had always struggled with his weight. He had tried every diet and exercise program out there, but nothing seemed to work. He would lose a few pounds, only to gain them back again. He was starting to lose hope that he would ever be able to achieve his weight loss goals.

One day, while browsing through a bookstore, John came across a book called "Weight Loss Affirmations." Intrigued, he picked it up and started reading. The book was filled with positive affirmations and motivational quotes designed to help people stay focused on their weight loss goals.

John was skeptical at first, but he decided to give the book a try. He started reading the affirmations every morning and every night before bed. At first, he didn't notice any changes. But slowly, he started to feel more motivated and encouraged.

He started making healthier choices when it came to food and exercise. He would repeat the affirmations to himself when he felt tempted to indulge in unhealthy snacks or skip a workout. And slowly but surely, he started to see results.

Over the course of several months, John lost over 50 pounds. He felt healthier and more confident than he had in years. And he knew that he had the "Weight Loss Affirmations" book to thank for helping him stay motivated and focused on his goals.

From that day forward, John made it a habit to read affirmations and motivational quotes every day. He knew that with the right mindset and attitude, he could achieve anything he set his mind to. And he was grateful for the book that had helped him realize that.

Welcome to "The Power of Weight Loss Affirmations"! This book is designed to help you achieve your weight loss goals through the power of positive affirmations. Losing weight can be a challenging journey, but with the right mindset and tools, it can be a rewarding one. In this book, we will explore the science behind affirmations and how they can help you overcome negative self-talk and limiting beliefs that may be holding you back from reaching your ideal weight. Through daily practice and repetition of these affirmations, you will develop a positive mindset that supports healthy habits and encourages self-love. Get ready to transform your relationship with food and your body as you embark on this empowering journey towards a healthier, happier you!

Chapter 1: Understand the power of affirmations for weight loss

Affirmations are powerful tools that can be used to help individuals achieve their weight loss goals. They are positive statements that are repeated to oneself in order to reinforce a particular belief or behavior. The power of affirmations lies in their ability to change the way we think and feel about ourselves, and ultimately, the actions we take.

One of the main reasons why affirmations work for weight loss is because they help to change our mindset. Many individuals who struggle with weight loss often have negative self-talk and beliefs about themselves. They may believe that they are not capable of losing weight, or that they do not deserve to have a healthy body.

Affirmations can help to counteract these negative beliefs by providing positive and empowering messages.

For example, an affirmation like "I am strong and capable of achieving my weight loss goals" can help to shift one's mindset from one of self-doubt to one of confidence and determination. Repeating this affirmation regularly can help to reinforce this new belief and motivate individuals to take action towards their weight loss goals.

Another way affirmations can help with weight loss is by promoting healthy behaviors. When individuals repeat affirmations related to healthy eating and exercise, they are more likely to make choices that align with those beliefs. For example, an affirmation like "I love nourishing my body with healthy foods" can help to reinforce the importance of healthy eating and encourage individuals to choose nutritious options over junk food.

In addition to promoting healthy behaviors, affirmations can also help to reduce stress and anxiety related to weight loss. Many individuals feel overwhelmed and discouraged when they do not see immediate results from their efforts. Affirmations can help to provide a sense of calm and reassurance, reminding individuals that they are making progress towards their goals and that they are capable of achieving them.

It is important to note that affirmations alone are not a magic solution for weight loss. They should be used in conjunction with healthy eating habits and regular exercise. However, incorporating affirmations into a weight loss plan can help to provide an additional layer of motivation and support.

Affirmations are a powerful tool that can be used to help individuals achieve their weight loss goals. They work by changing our mindset, promoting healthy behaviors, and reducing stress and anxiety related to weight loss. By incorporating affirmations into a weight loss plan, individuals can increase their chances of success and achieve a healthier, happier, and more confident version of themselves.

chapter 2: Creating an Affirmation Practice

Creating an affirmation practice is an important step in using affirmations for weight loss. Here are some pointers to get you going:

1. Set aside time each day: Choose a specific time of day when you can focus on your affirmations without distractions. This might be done first thing in the morning, during lunch, or right before bed.

2. Find a quiet space: Choose a quiet space where you can sit or stand comfortably without interruptions. This might be a corner of your bedroom, a peaceful park, or a quiet room in your home.

3. Choose your affirmations: Select affirmations that resonate with you and support your weight loss goals. Write them down or record them on your phone so you can easily access them during your affirmation practice.

4. Repeat your affirmations: Repeat your affirmations out loud or silently to yourself. Focus on the meaning behind each affirmation and visualize yourself achieving your goals.

5. Use visualization techniques: As you repeat your affirmations, use visualization techniques to imagine yourself achieving your weight loss goals. Visualize yourself feeling healthy, energized, and confident in your body.

6. Be consistent: Consistency is key when it comes to affirmations. Make a commitment to repeat your affirmations daily, even if it's just for a few minutes each day.

By creating an affirmation practice, you can harness the power of positive thinking to support your weight loss goals. With regular practice, you'll begin to shift your mindset and behaviors around food and exercise, making it easier to achieve lasting weight loss success.

Chapter 3: Affirmations for healthy eating habits

When it comes to healthy eating habits, affirmations can be a powerful tool to help shift your mindset and behaviors around food. Below are some affirmations to help support your journey towards healthier eating habits:

1. I choose to nourish my body with healthy and nutritious foods.

2. I am in control of my food choices and make choices that support my health and wellbeing.

3. I listen to my body's hunger and fullness cues and eat mindfully.

4. I am grateful for the abundance of healthy food options available to me.

5. I enjoy preparing and cooking healthy meals for myself and my loved ones.

6. I choose to eat foods that fuel my body with energy and vitality.

7. I am worthy of taking care of my body through healthy eating habits.

8. I honor my body by choosing foods that make me feel good from the inside out.

9. I let go of guilt and shame around food choices and instead focus on nourishment and balance.

10. I trust myself to make healthy food choices that support my goals.

11. I am grateful for the positive changes that healthy eating habits bring into my life.

12. I choose to eat mindfully and savor each bite of food.

13. I am patient with myself as I develop healthier eating habits.

14. I release any negative thoughts or beliefs around food and embrace a positive and nourishing mindset.

15. I am excited to explore new healthy foods and recipes that support my health goals.

16. I prioritize self-care by choosing healthy foods that support my physical, emotional, and mental wellbeing.

17. I trust my body's signals and stop eating when I am satisfied.

18. I choose to be kind to myself and give myself grace when it comes to healthy eating habits.

19. I am proud of myself for making positive changes towards healthier eating habits.

20. I am committed to making healthy eating habits a sustainable and enjoyable part of my life.

Chapter 4: Affirmations for exercise and physical activity

Regular exercise and physical activity are essential for maintaining good health and wellbeing. Here are 20 affirmations to help motivate and inspire you to incorporate exercise into your daily routine:

1. I am committed to making exercise a priority in my life.

2. I am capable of achieving my fitness goals through consistent effort and dedication.

3. I enjoy moving my body and challenging myself with new exercises and activities.

4. I am grateful for the physical strength and endurance that exercise provides me.

5. I trust my body's ability to adapt and improve with regular exercise.

6. I am worthy of taking care of my body through regular physical activity.

7. I listen to my body's signals and adjust my workouts accordingly.

8. I am proud of myself for making time for exercise in my busy schedule.

9. I choose to focus on the positive benefits of exercise, such as increased energy and improved mood.

10. I am patient with myself as I work towards my fitness goals.

11. I am grateful for the supportive community of people who encourage me to stay active and healthy.

12. I embrace the challenge of pushing myself beyond my comfort zone during workouts.

13. I release any negative thoughts or beliefs about exercise and embrace a positive and empowering mindset.

14. I am excited to see the progress and improvements in my physical abilities with consistent exercise.

15. I prioritize self-care by making time for exercise and physical activity in my daily routine.

16. I trust the process of gradual improvement and celebrate each small victory along the way.

17. I choose to make exercise a fun and enjoyable part of my daily life.

18. I am proud of myself for showing up and putting in the effort towards my fitness goals.

19. I am grateful for the opportunity to move my body and feel alive.

20. I am committed to making exercise a sustainable and lifelong habit for my health and wellbeing.

Chapter 5: Affirmations for Positive Body Image and Self-Love

It's important to practice self-love and acceptance when it comes to our bodies. Here are 20 affirmations to help you cultivate a positive body image and love yourself just the way you are:

1. I love and accept myself exactly as I am.

2. My body is unique and beautiful in its own way.

3. I choose to focus on what my body can do rather than its appearance.

4. I am grateful for all the amazing things my body does for me every day.

5. I trust my body's natural ability to heal and regenerate itself.

6. I am worthy of love and respect regardless of my size or shape.

7. I release any negative thoughts or beliefs about my body and embrace a positive and empowering mindset.

8. I choose to nourish my body with healthy foods and exercise because it feels good, not because I want to change its appearance.

9. I am proud of my body and all the challenges it has overcome.

10. I am grateful for the supportive people in my life who love and accept me just the way I am.

11. I choose to surround myself with positive and uplifting messages that reinforce my self-love and acceptance.

12. I am confident in my own skin and radiate that confidence to others.

13. I honor my body's needs and listen to its signals for rest, nourishment, and movement.

14. I am deserving of self-care and prioritize it in my daily routine.

15. I choose to let go of comparison and embrace my own unique beauty.
16. I am grateful for the gift of life and appreciate my body for all that it does to keep me alive and thriving.

17. I trust that my body knows what's best for me and will guide me towards optimal health and wellbeing.

18. I am proud of myself for working towards a positive body image and self-love.

19. I choose to celebrate my body and all its imperfections because they make me who I am.

20. I am committed to practicing self-love and acceptance every day, for the rest of my life.

Chapter 6: Affirmations for Overcoming Emotional Eating and Cravings

Emotional eating and cravings can be a challenge, but it's important to remember that we have the power to overcome them. Here are 20 affirmations to help you break free from emotional eating and cravings:

1. I am in control of my eating habits and choose to nourish my body with healthy foods.

2. I trust my body's signals for hunger and fullness and honor them accordingly.

3. I release any guilt or shame associated with emotional eating and forgive myself for past mistakes.

4. I choose to address the root cause of my emotional eating and work towards healing those issues.

5. I am worthy of self-love and care, even when I struggle with emotional eating.

6. I am capable of overcoming my cravings and choosing healthier options.

7. I choose to focus on the positive changes I'm making rather than dwelling on past mistakes.

8. I am grateful for the opportunity to learn and grow from my experiences with emotional eating.

9. I choose to listen to my body's needs and give it what it truly craves, whether that be rest, movement, or nourishing foods.

10. I am proud of myself for taking steps towards a healthier relationship with food.

11. I am deserving of a life free from the negative effects of emotional eating.

12. I trust that my body knows what's best for me and will guide me towards optimal health and wellbeing.

13. I choose to let go of any negative self-talk or limiting beliefs that hold me back from achieving my goals.

14. I am committed to practicing self-care and self-love every day, even when it's difficult.

15. I am capable of finding healthy ways to cope with my emotions without turning to food.

16. I am grateful for the support of loved ones who encourage me on my journey towards a healthier lifestyle.

17. I choose to celebrate my progress and small victories along the way.

18. I am proud of myself for making positive changes in my life and breaking free from emotional eating.

19. I am worthy of a life filled with joy, happiness, and freedom from emotional eating.

20. I trust that with time, patience, and self-love, I will overcome my struggles with emotional eating and cravings.

Chapter 7: Affirmations for Stress Management and Mindful Eating

Stress can often lead to mindless eating, but it's important to remember that we can manage our stress and practice mindful eating. Here are 20 affirmations to help you manage stress and eat mindfully:

1. I am in control of my stress levels and choose to prioritize self-care.

2. I trust my body's signals for hunger and fullness and honor them accordingly.

3. I release any guilt or shame associated with mindless eating and forgive myself for past mistakes.

4. I choose to address the root cause of my stress and work towards managing those issues.

5. I am worthy of self-love and care, even when I struggle with mindless eating.

6. I am capable of overcoming my stress and choosing healthier options.

7. I choose to focus on the present moment and be mindful of my eating habits.

8. I am grateful for the opportunity to learn and grow from my experiences with stress and mindless eating.

9. I choose to listen to my body's needs and give it what it truly craves, whether that be rest, movement, or nourishing foods.

10. I am proud of myself for taking steps towards a healthier relationship with food and managing stress.

11. I am deserving of a life free from the negative effects of stress and mindless eating.

12. I trust that my body knows what's best for me and will guide me towards optimal health and wellbeing.

13. I choose to let go of any negative self-talk or limiting beliefs that hold me back from achieving my goals.

14. I am committed to practicing mindfulness in all aspects of my life, including eating.

15. I am capable of finding healthy ways to cope with my stress without turning to food.

16. I am grateful for the support of loved ones who encourage me on my journey towards a healthier lifestyle.

17. I choose to celebrate my progress and small victories along the way.

18. I am proud of myself for making positive changes in my life and breaking free from mindless eating and stress.

19. I am worthy of a life filled with joy, happiness, and freedom from stress and mindless eating.

20. I trust that with time, patience, and self-love, I will overcome my struggles with stress and mindless eating and live a fulfilling life.

Chapter 8: Affirmations for Consistency and Motivation

Consistency and motivation are key to achieving any goal, including maintaining a healthy lifestyle. Here are 20 affirmations to help you stay consistent and motivated on your journey towards optimal health and wellbeing:

1. I am committed to making positive changes in my life and will remain consistent in my efforts.

2. I trust that every small step I take towards my goals will lead to significant progress over time.

3. I choose to focus on the present moment and take action towards my goals every day.

4. I am worthy of achieving my goals and will not give up, no matter how challenging the journey may be.

5. I am capable of overcoming any obstacles that come my way and staying consistent in my efforts.

6. I choose to prioritize self-care and make time for activities that bring me joy and fulfillment.

7. I am grateful for the progress I've made so far and will use it as motivation to continue moving forward.

8. I trust that with consistency, dedication, and hard work, I will achieve my desired results.

9. I am proud of myself for taking ownership of my health and making positive changes in my life.

10. I choose to surround myself with positivity and encouragement, whether it be through loved ones or affirmations.

11. I am deserving of a life filled with health, happiness, and vitality, and will remain consistent in my efforts to achieve it.

12. I trust that my body is capable of achieving optimal health and will work towards nourishing it with healthy habits.

13. I choose to celebrate my progress, no matter how small, and use it as motivation to keep going.

14. I am grateful for the opportunity to learn and grow from my experiences, both positive and negative.

15. I am capable of finding balance in my life and maintaining consistency in my healthy habits.

16. I choose to let go of any negative self-talk or limiting beliefs that hold me back from achieving my goals.

17. I am proud of myself for taking responsibility for my health and wellbeing and making positive changes in my life.

18. I am committed to staying consistent in my efforts, even when faced with challenges or setbacks.

19. I trust that my consistency and motivation will lead to a happier, healthier, and more fulfilling life.

20. I am capable of achieving my goals and will remain consistent and motivated on my journey towards optimal health and wellbeing.

Chapter 9: Affirmations for Dealing with Plateaus and Setbacks

Plateaus and setbacks are a natural part of any journey towards optimal health and wellbeing. Here are 20 affirmations to help you stay positive and motivated during times of stagnation or setbacks:

1. I trust that plateaus and setbacks are temporary and will not derail my progress towards my goals.

2. I choose to view plateaus and setbacks as opportunities for growth and learning.

3. I am capable of overcoming any obstacles that come my way, including plateaus and setbacks.

4. I am grateful for the progress I've made so far and will use it as motivation to continue moving forward.

5. I trust that with patience, persistence, and hard work, I will overcome any plateau or setback.

6. I choose to focus on the present moment and take action towards my goals every day, regardless of any setbacks.

7. I am worthy of achieving my goals and will not give up, no matter how challenging the journey may be.

8. I am proud of myself for taking ownership of my health and making positive changes in my life, even in the face of setbacks.

9. I choose to surround myself with positivity and encouragement, whether it be through loved ones or affirmations.

10. I am deserving of a life filled with health, happiness, and vitality, and will remain consistent in my efforts to achieve it.

11. I trust that my body is capable of achieving optimal health, even in the face of plateaus and setbacks.

12. I choose to celebrate my progress, no matter how small, and use it as motivation to keep going.

13. I am grateful for the opportunity to learn and grow from my experiences, both positive and negative.

14. I am capable of finding new strategies and approaches to overcome plateaus and setbacks.

15. I choose to let go of any negative self-talk or limiting beliefs that hold me back from overcoming plateaus and setbacks.

16. I am proud of myself for taking responsibility for my health and wellbeing and making positive changes in my life, even in the face of setbacks.

17. I am committed to staying consistent in my efforts, even when faced with plateaus or setbacks.

18. I trust that my consistency and motivation will lead to a happier, healthier, and more fulfilling life, even in the face of setbacks.

19. I am capable of achieving my goals, even if it takes longer than expected due to plateaus or setbacks.

20. I choose to remain positive and focused on my goals, knowing that every setback is an opportunity for growth and learning.

Conclusion and next steps:

Plateaus and setbacks are a natural part of any journey towards optimal health and wellbeing. It's important to remember that these challenges are temporary and can be overcome with persistence, patience, and hard work. By incorporating these affirmations into your daily routine, you can stay positive and motivated even in the face of adversity.

Moving forward, it's important to remain consistent in your efforts and surround yourself with positivity and encouragement. Take time to celebrate your progress, no matter how small, and use it as motivation to keep going. Remember that every setback is an opportunity for growth and learning, so don't give up on your goals.

In addition to using affirmations, consider seeking support from loved ones or a healthcare professional. They can provide guidance, encouragement, and accountability to help you stay on track and overcome any challenges that come your way.

By staying committed to your goals and using positive affirmations, you can achieve a happier, healthier, and more fulfilling life. Keep pushing forward, and never give up on your journey towards optimal health and wellbeing.